The Comprehensive Plant-Based Recipe Book

50 Super Easy Plant-Based Recipes You'll Want to Make Everyday

Levi Tonge

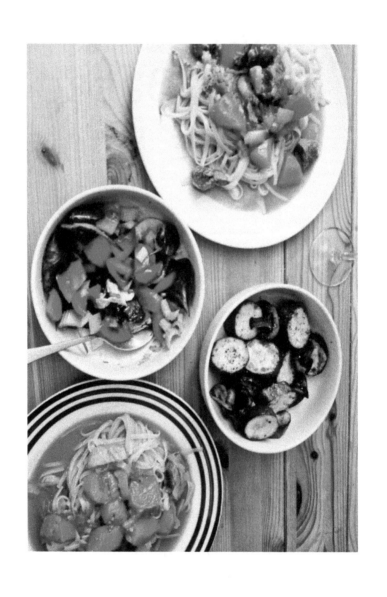

advice. The content within this book has been derived from various sources. Please consult a licensed professional before attempting any techniques outlined in this book.

By reading this document, the reader agrees that under no circumstances is the author responsible for any losses, direct or indirect, which are incurred as a result of the use of information contained within this document, including, but not limited to, — errors, omissions, or inaccuracies.

Table of Contents

White Bean and Walnut Patties

Servings: 4

Cooking Time: 7 Minutes

Ingredients:

- ¼ cup diced onion
- 1 garlic clove, crushed
- ¾ cup walnut pieces
- ¾ cup canned or cooked white beans, drained and rinsed
- ¾ cup wheat gluten flour (vital wheat gluten)
- 2 tablespoons minced fresh parsley
- 1 tablespoon soy sauce
- 1 teaspoon Dijon mustard, plus more to serve
- ½ teaspoon salt
- ½ teaspoon ground sage
- ½ teaspoon sweet paprika
- ¼ teaspoon turmeric
- ¼ teaspoon freshly ground black pepper
- 2 tablespoons extra-virgin olive oil
- Bread or rolls of choice
- Lettuce leaves and sliced tomatoes

Directions:

1.   Preparing the Ingredients

2.   In a food processor, combine the onion, garlic, and walnuts, then process until finely ground.

3.   Cook the beans in a small skillet over medium heat, stirring, for 1 - 2 minutes to evaporate any moisture. Add the beans to the food processor along with the flour, parsley, soy sauce, mustard, salt, sage, paprika, turmeric, and pepper. Process until well blended. Shape the mixture into 4 equal patties.

4.   Cook

5.   In a large skillet, heat the oil over medium heat. Add the patties and cook until browned on both sides, about minutes per side.

6.   Finish and Serve

7.   Serve on your favorite sandwich bread with mustard, lettuce, and sliced tomatoes.

Black Bean and Corn Salad with Cilantro Dressing
Servings: 4

Cooking Time: 0 Minutes

Ingredients:

- 2 cups frozen corn, thawed
- 3 cups cooked or 2 (15.5-ounce) cans black beans, rinsed and drained
- ½ cup chopped red bell pepper
- ¼ cup minced red onion
- 1 (4-ounce) can chopped mild green chiles, drained
- 2 garlic cloves, crushed
- ¼ cup chopped fresh cilantro
- 1 teaspoon ground cumin
- ½ teaspoon salt (optional)
- ¼ teaspoon freshly ground black pepper
- 2 tablespoons fresh lime juice
- 2 tablespoons water
- ¼ cup extra-virgin olive oil

Directions:

1. Preparing the Ingredients
2. In a large bowl, combine the corn, beans, bell pepper, onion, and chiles. Set aside.

3.   In a blender or food processor, mince the garlic. Add the cilantro, cumin, salt, and black pepper, then pulse to blend. Add the lime juice, water, and oil and process until well blended.

4.   Finish and Serve

5.   Pour the dressing over the salad and toss to combine. Taste and adjust the seasonings if necessary, then serve.

Stuffed Peppers

Servings: 4

Cooking Time: 20 Minutes

Ingredients:

- 2 green onions, sliced
- 2 green bell peppers, halved, cored
- 1 large tomato, diced
- 1/2 cup Arborio rice, cooked
- ¼ teaspoon ground black pepper
- 1 teaspoon Italian seasoning
- 1 teaspoon salt
- 1 teaspoon dried basil
- 1 tablespoon olive oil
- 1 cup of water
- 1/2 cup crumbled vegan feta cheese

Directions:

1.   Prepare the peppers and for this, cut them in half, then remove the seeds and roast them on a greased baking sheet for 20 minutes at 400 degrees F until tender.

2.   Meanwhile, heat oil in a skillet pan over medium-high heat and when hot, add onion, season with seasonings and herbs, and cook for 3 minutes.

3.   Add tomatoes, stir well, cook for 5 minutes, then stir in rice and cook for minutes until heated.

4.   When done, remove the pan from heat, stir in cheese, and stuff the mixture into roasted peppers.

5.   Serve straight away.

Nutrition Info: Calories: 385 Cal; Fat: 15.2 g: Carbs: 52.6 g; Protein: 10.8 g; Fiber: 4.5 g

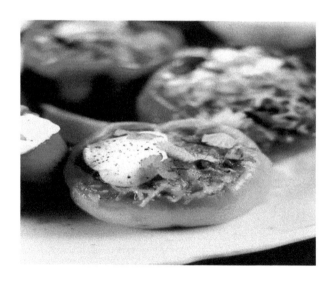

Brown Rice and Lentil Pilaf
Servings: 4 To 6

Cooking Time: 50 Minutes

Ingredients:
- 1 tablespoon extra-virgin olive oil
- 1 large yellow onion, minced
- 1 medium carrot, chopped
- 2 garlic cloves, minced
- 1 cup long-grain brown rice
- 1½ teaspoons ground coriander
- ½ teaspoon ground cumin
- 3 cups water
- Salt
- 3 tablespoons minced fresh cilantro
- Freshly ground black pepper

Directions:
1. Preparing the Ingredients
2. Bring a saucepan of salted water to boil over high heat. Add the lentils, return to a boil, then reduce heat to medium and cook for 15 minutes. Drain and set aside. In a large saucepan, heat the oil over medium heat. Add

the onion, carrot, and garlic, cover, then cook until tender for about 10 minutes.

3.   Add the lentils to the vegetable mixture. Add the rice, coriander, and cumin. Stir in the water and bring to boil. Reduce heat to low, salt the water, and cook, covered, until the lentils and rice are tender for about minutes.

4.   Finish and Serve

5.   Remove from heat and set aside for 10 minutes.

6.   Transfer to a large bowl, fluff with a fork, then sprinkle with the cilantro and freshly ground black pepper. Serve immediately.

Chickpea And Vegetable Loaf

Servings: 4

Cooking Time: 10 Minutes

Ingredients:

- 1 small white potato, peeled and shredded
- 1 medium carrot, shredded
- 1 small yellow onion, chopped
- 2 garlic cloves, minced
- 1½ cups cooked or 1 (15.5-ounce) can chickpeas, drained and rinsed
- ¾ cup wheat gluten flour or chickpea flour, or more if needed
- ¾ cup quick-cooking oats
- ½ cup dry unseasoned bread crumbs
- ¼ cup minced fresh parsley
- 1 tablespoon soy sauce
- 1 teaspoon dried savory
- ½ teaspoon dried sage
- 1 teaspoon salt
- ¼ teaspoon freshly ground black pepper

Directions:

1. Preparing the Ingredients

2.　　Preheat the oven to 350°F. Lightly oil a 9-inch loaf pan and set aside. Squeeze the excess liquid from the shredded potato and place it in a food processor, along with the carrot, onion, and garlic. Add the chickpeas and pulse to blend the Ingredients while retaining some texture. Add the flour, oats, bread crumbs, parsley, soy sauce, savory, sage, salt, and black pepper. Pulse just until blended.

3.　　Scrape the mixture onto a lightly floured work surface. Use your hands to form the mixture into a loaf, adding more flour or oats if the mixture is too loose.

4.　　Bake

5.　　Place the loaf in the prepared pan, smoothing the top. Bake until firm and golden, about 1 hour.

6.　　Remove from oven and let stand for 10 minutes before slicing.

Lentil, Rice and Vegetable Bake
Servings: 6

Cooking Time: 40 Minutes

Ingredients:

- 1/2 cup white rice, cooked
- 1 cup red lentils, cooked
- 1/3 cup chopped carrots
- 1 medium tomato, chopped
- 1 small onion, peeled, chopped
- 1/3 cup chopped zucchini
- 1/3 cup chopped celery
- 1 ½ teaspoon minced garlic
- ½ teaspoon ground black pepper
- 1 teaspoon dried basil
- 1 teaspoon ground cumin
- 1 teaspoon dried oregano
- ½ teaspoon salt
- 1 teaspoon olive oil
- 8 ounces tomato sauce

Directions:

1.   Take a skillet pan, place it over medium heat, add oil and when hot, add onion and garlic, and cook for 5 minutes.

2.   Then add remaining vegetables, season with salt, black pepper, and half of each cumin, oregano and basil and cook for 5 minutes until vegetables are tender.

3.   Take a casserole dish, place lentils and rice in it, top with vegetables, spread with tomato sauce and sprinkle with remaining cumin, oregano, and basil, and bake for minutes until bubbly.

4.   Serve straight away.

Nutrition Info: Calories: 187 Cal; Fat: 1.5 g: Carbs: 35.1 g; Protein: 9.7 g; Fiber: 8.1 g

Vegan Curried Rice

Servings: 4

Cooking Time: 25 Minutes

Ingredients:

- 1 cup white rice
- 1 tablespoon minced garlic
- 1 tablespoon ground curry powder
- 1/3 teaspoon ground black pepper
- 1 tablespoon red chili powder
- 1 tablespoon ground cumin
- 2 tablespoons olive oil
- 1 tablespoon soy sauce
- 1 cup vegetable broth

Directions:

1.   Take a saucepan, place it over low heat, add oil and when hot, add garlic and cook for 3 minutes.

2.   Then stir in all spices, cook for 1 minute until fragrant, pour in the broth, and switch heat to a high level.

3.   Stir in soy sauce, bring the mixture to boil, add rice, stir until mixed, then switch heat to the low level

and simmer for 20 minutes until rice is tender and all the liquid has absorbed.

4.   Serve straight away.

Nutrition Info: Calories: 262 Cal; Fat: 8 g: Carbs: 43 g; Protein: 5 g; Fiber: 2 g

Jerk-spiced Red Bean Chili

Servings: 4

Cooking Time: 50 Minutes

Ingredients:

- 1 tablespoon extra-virgin olive oil
- 1 medium onion, chopped
- 8 ounces seitan, chopped
- 3 cups cooked or 2 (15.5-ounce) cans dark red kidney beans, drained and rinsed
- 1 (14.5-ounce) can crushed tomatoes
- 1 (14.5-ounce) can diced tomatoes, drained
- 1 (4-ounce) can chopped mild or hot green chiles, drained
- ½ cup barbecue sauce
- 1 cup water
- 1 tablespoon soy sauce
- 1 tablespoon chili powder
- 1 teaspoon ground cumin
- 1 teaspoon ground allspice
- ½ teaspoon ground oregano
- ¼ teaspoon ground cayenne
- ½ teaspoon salt
- ¼ teaspoon freshly ground black pepper

Directions:

1.   Preparing the Ingredients

2.   In a large pot, heat the oil over medium heat. Add the onion and seitan. Cover and cook until the onion is softened for about 10 minutes.

3.   Stir in the kidney beans, crushed tomatoes, diced tomatoes, and chiles. Stir in the barbecue sauce, water, soy sauce, chili powder, cumin, allspice, sugar, oregano, cayenne, salt, and black pepper.

4.   Bring to boil, then reduce the heat to medium and simmer, covered, until the vegetables are tender for about minutes.

5.   Finish and Serve

6.   Uncover and simmer about 10 minutes longer. Serve immediately.

Chickpea and Artichoke Curry

Servings: 4

Cooking Time: 15 Minutes

Ingredients:

- 1 teaspoon extra-virgin olive oil or 2 teaspoons vegetable broth
- 1 small onion, diced
- 2 teaspoons minced garlic (2 cloves)
- 1 (14.5-ounce) can chickpeas, rinsed and drained
- 1 (14.5-ounce) can artichoke hearts, drained and quartered
- 2 teaspoons curry powder
- ½ teaspoon ground coriander
- ½ teaspoon ground cumin
- 1 (5.4-ounce) can unsweetened coconut milk

Directions:

1. Preparing the Ingredients.

2. In a large skillet or pot over medium-high heat, heat the olive oil. Add the onion and garlic and sauté for about 5 minutes. Add the chickpeas, artichoke hearts, curry powder, coriander, and cumin. Stir to combine well.

3.   Pour the coconut milk into the pot, mix well, and bring to a boil. Cover, reduce the heat to low, and simmer for 10 minutes.

4.   Divide the curry evenly among wide-mouth glass jars or single-compartment containers. Let cool before sealing the lids.

Nutrition Info: Per Serving: Calories: 267; Fat: 12g; Protein: 9g; Carbohydrates: 36g; Fiber: 11g; Sugar: 3g; Sodium: 373mg

Coconut Curry Lentils

Servings: 4

Cooking Time: 40 Minutes

Ingredients:

- 1 cup brown lentils
- 1 small white onion, peeled, chopped
- 1 teaspoon minced garlic
- 1 teaspoon grated ginger
- 3 cups baby spinach
- 1 tablespoon curry powder
- 2 tablespoons olive oil
- 13 ounces coconut milk, unsweetened
- 2 cups vegetable broth
- For Serving:
- 4 cups cooked rice
- 1/4 cup chopped cilantro

Directions:

1. Place a large pot over medium heat, add oil and when hot, add ginger and garlic and cook for minute until fragrant.

2.   Add onion, cook for 5 minutes, stir in curry powder, cook for 1 minute until toasted, add lentils and pour in broth.

3.   Switch heat to medium-high level, bring the mixture to a boil, then switch heat to the low level and simmer for 20 minutes until tender and all the liquid is absorbed.

4.   Pour in milk, stir until combined, turn heat to medium level, and simmer for 10 minutes until thickened.

5.   Then remove the pot from heat, stir in spinach, let it stand for minutes until its leaves wilts and then top with cilantro.

6.   Serve lentils with rice.

Nutrition Info: Calories: 184 Cal; Fat: 3.7 g: Carbs: 30 g; Protein: 11.3 g; Fiber: 10.7 g

Cinnamon Chickpeas (pressure Cooker)

Servings: 4-6

Cooking Time: 12 Minutes

Ingredients:

- 1 cup dried chickpeas, soaked in water overnight
- 2 cups water
- 2 teaspoons ground cinnamon, plus more as needed
- ½ teaspoon ground nutmeg (optional)
- 1 tablespoon coconut oil
- 2 to 4 tablespoons unrefined sugar or brown sugar, plus more as needed

Directions:

1. Preparing the Ingredients. Drain and rinse the chickpeas, then put them in your electric pressure cooker's cooking pot. Add the water, cinnamon, and nutmeg (if using).

2. High pressure for 30 minutes. Lock the lid and ensure the pressure valve is sealed, then select High Pressure and set the time for 30 minutes.

3. Pressure Release. Once the cook time is complete, let the pressure release naturally for about 15 minutes.

Once all the pressure has released, unlock and remove the lid. Drain any excess water from the chickpeas and add them back to the pot. Stir in the coconut oil and sugar. Taste and add more cinnamon, if desired.

4.	Select Sauté and cook for about 5 minutes, stirring the chickpeas occasionally, until there's no liquid left and the sugar has melted onto the chickpeas. Transfer to a bowl and toss with additional sugar if you want to add a crunchy texture.

Nutrition Info: Per Serving: Calories 253; Total fat: 7g; Protein: 11g; Sodium: 9mg; Fiber: 10g

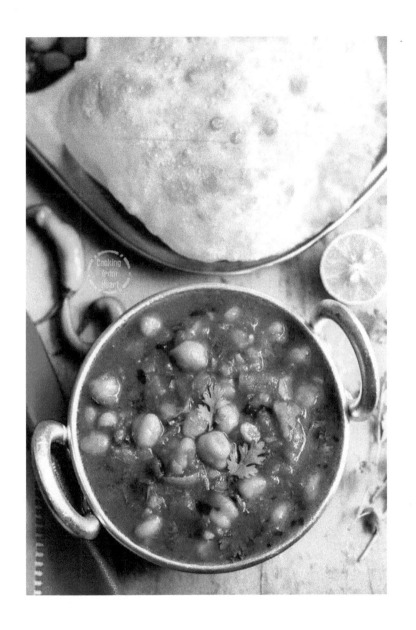

Brown Rice with Artichokes, Chickpeas, and Tomatoes

Servings: 4

Cooking Time: 30 Minutes

Ingredients:

- 2 tablespoons extra-virgin olive oil
- 3 garlic cloves, minced
- 1 cup frozen artichokes hearts, thawed and chopped
- 1 teaspoon dried basil
- ½teaspoon dried marjoram
- 1½ cups cooked or 1 (15.5-ounce) can chickpeas, drained and rinsed
- 1½ cups long-grain brown rice
- 3 cups vegetable broth
- Salt and freshly ground black pepper
- 1 cup ripe grape tomatoes, quartered
- 2 tablespoons minced fresh parsley

Directions:

1. Preparing the Ingredients

2. In a large saucepan, heat the oil over medium heat. Add the garlic and cook until softened for about 1 minute. Add the artichokes, basil, marjoram, and

chickpeas. Stir in the rice and broth. Season with salt and pepper.

3.   Cover tightly and reduce heat to low. Simmer until the rice is cooked for about minutes.

4.   Finish and Serve

5.   Transfer to a serving bowl, add the tomatoes and parsley, taste and adjust seasonings if necessary, then fluff with a fork. Serve immediately.

Brown Rice and Lentils
Servings: 4

Cooking Time: 15 Minutes

Ingredients:

- 2 tablespoons extra-virgin olive oil
- 1 onion, diced
- 1 carrot, diced
- 1 celery stalk, diced
- two 15-ounce cans lentils, drained and rinsed
- one 15-ounce can diced tomatoes with juice
- 1 tablespoon dried rosemary
- 1 tablespoon garlic powder
- 2 cups prepared brown rice
- sea salt
- freshly ground black pepper

Directions:

1. Preparing the Ingredients

2. In a large pot, heat the olive oil over medium-high heat until it shimmers.

3. Add the onion, carrot, and celery and cook until the vegetables soften. Add the lentils, tomatoes,

rosemary, and garlic powder. Lower the heat to medium-low and simmer to blend the flavors for 5 to 7 minutes.

4.   Finish and Serve

5.   Stir the rice into lentils and heat through for 2 to 3 minutes. Season with salt and pepper, then serve immediately.

Black Beans and Rice

Servings: 4

Cooking Time: 30 Minutes

Ingredients:

- 3/4 cup white rice
- 1 medium white onion, peeled, chopped
- 3 1/2 cups cooked black beans
- 1 teaspoon minced garlic
- 1/4 teaspoon cayenne pepper
- 1 teaspoon ground cumin
- 1 teaspoon olive oil
- 1 1/2 cups vegetable broth

Directions:

1.   Take a large pot over medium-high heat, add oil and when hot, add onion and garlic and cook for 4 minutes until saute.

2.   Then stir in rice, cook for minutes, pour in the broth, bring it to a boil, switch heat to the low level and cook for 20 minutes until tender.

3.   Stir in remaining ingredients, cook for 2 minutes, and then serve straight away.

Nutrition Info: Calories: 140 Cal; Fat: 0.9 g: Carbs: 27.1 g; Protein: 6.3 g; Fiber: 6.2 g

Chinese Black Bean Chili

Servings: 4

Cooking Time: 0 Minutes

Ingredients:

- 1 tablespoon extra-virgin olive oil
- 1 medium yellow onion, finely chopped
- 2 medium carrots, finely chopped
- 1 teaspoon grated fresh ginger
- 2 tablespoons chili powder
- 1 teaspoon brown sugar
- 1 (28-ounce) can diced tomatoes, undrained
- ½ cup Chinese black bean sauce
- ¾ cup water
- 4½ cups cooked or 3 (15.5-ounce) cans black beans, drained and rinsed
- Salt and freshly ground black pepper
- 2 tablespoons minced green onion, for garnish

Directions:

1. Preparing the Ingredients
2. In a large pot, heat the oil over medium heat. Add the onion and carrot. Cover and cook until softened for about 10 minutes.

3.   Stir in the ginger, chili powder, and sugar. Add the tomatoes, black bean sauce, and water. Stir in the black beans and season with salt and pepper.

4.   Bring to boil, then reduce the heat to medium and simmer, covered, until the vegetables are tender for about 30 minutes.

5.   Finish and Serve

6.   Simmer for about 10 minutes longer. Serve immediately garnished with green onion.

Three Lentil Dal

Servings: 6

Cooking Time: 65 Minutes

Ingredients:

- ½ cup green lentils, picked over, rinsed, and drained
- ½ cup brown lentils, picked over, rinsed, and drained
- 3 cups water
- Salt
- ½ cup red lentils, picked over, rinsed, and drained
- 2 tablespoons canola or grapeseed oil
- 1 medium yellow onion, minced
- 2 garlic cloves, minced
- 2 teaspoons grated fresh ginger
- 1 tablespoon hot or mild curry powder
- ½ teaspoon ground cumin
- ½ teaspoon ground coriander
- ¼ teaspoon ground cayenne
- 1 (14.5-ounce) can crushed tomatoes

Directions:

1. Preparing the Ingredients

2.   Soak the green lentils and brown lentils in separate medium bowls of hot water for 45 minutes. Drain the green lentils and place them in a large saucepan with the water. Bring to boil. Reduce heat to low and simmer for 10 minutes.

3.   Drain the brown lentils and add to the green lentils with salt. Simmer partially covered for 20 minutes while stirring occasionally. Add the red lentils and simmer, uncovered, until the sauce thickens and the beans are very soft for 20 to 25 minutes longer.

4.   In a large skillet, heat the oil over medium heat. Add the onion, cover, and cook until softened for about 10 minutes. Add the garlic and ginger and cook until fragrant.

5.   Finish and Serve

6.   Add the curry powder, cumin, coriander, cayenne, and tomatoes, stirring constantly for about 1 minute. Add the tomato mixture to the cooked lentils and stir to mix well. Cook for another 10 minutes until the flavors are blended. Taste and adjust the seasonings if necessary. Serve immediately.

Lentil And Wild Rice Soup

Servings: 4

Cooking Time: 40 Minutes

Ingredients:

- 1/2 cup cooked mixed beans
- 12 ounces cooked lentils
- 2 stalks of celery, sliced
- 1 1/2 cup mixed wild rice, cooked
- 1 large sweet potato, peeled, chopped
- 1/2 medium butternut, peeled, chopped
- 4 medium carrots, peeled, sliced
- 1 medium onion, peeled, diced
- 10 cherry tomatoes
- 1/2 red chili, deseeded, diced
- 1 ½ teaspoon minced garlic
- 1/2 teaspoon salt
- 2 teaspoons mixed dried herbs
- 1 teaspoon coconut oil
- 2 cups vegetable broth

Directions:

1.   Take a large pot, place it over medium-high heat, add oil and when it melts, add onion and cook for 5 minutes.

2.   Stir in garlic and chili, cook for 3 minutes, then add remaining vegetables, pour in the broth, stir and bring the mixture to a boil.

3.   Switch heat to medium-low heat, cook the soup for 20 minutes, then stir in remaining ingredients and continue cooking for 10 minutes until soup has reached to desired thickness.

4.   Serve straight away.

Nutrition Info: Calories: 331 Cal; Fat: 2 g: Carbs: 54 g; Protein: 13 g; Fiber: 12 g

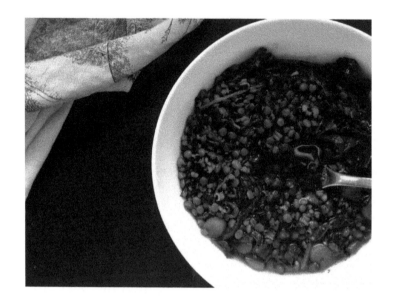

Green Tea Rice with Lemon Snow Peas and Tofu

Servings: 4

Cooking Time: 30 Minutes

Ingredients:

- 3 cups water
- 4 green tea bags
- 1½ cups white sushi rice
- 2 tablespoons canola or grapeseed oil
- 8 ounces extra-firm tofu, drained and cut into 1/4-inch dice
- 3 green onions, minced
- 2 cups snow peas, trimmed and cut diagonally into 1-inch pieces
- 1 tablespoon fresh lemon juice
- 1 teaspoon grated lemon zest
- Salt and freshly ground black pepper

Directions:

1. Preparing the Ingredients
2. In a large saucepan, bring the water to a boil. Add the tea bags and remove from the heat. Let stand for 7 minutes and remove and discard the tea bags. Rinse the

rice under running water until the water runs clear, then add to the brewed tea.

3.   Cook

4.   Cover and cook over medium heat until tender, about 25 minutes. Remove from heat and set aside.

5.   In a large skillet, heat the oil over medium heat. Add the tofu and cook until golden brown, minutes. Add the green onions and snow peas and cook until softened, 3 minutes. Stir in the lemon juice and zest.

6.   In a large bowl, combine the cooked rice with the tofu and snow pea mixture.

7.   Finish and Serve

8.   Season with salt and pepper to taste, and serve immediately.

Grilled Ahlt

Servings: 1

Cooking Time: 10 Minutes

Ingredients:

- ¼ cup Classic Hummus
- 2 slices whole-grain bread
- ¼ avocado, sliced
- ½ cup lettuce, chopped
- ½ tomato, sliced
- Pinch sea salt
- Pinch freshly ground black pepper
- 1 teaspoon extra-virgin olive oil divided

Directions:

1.	Preparing the Ingredients

2.	Spread some hummus on each slice of bread. Then layer the avocado, lettuce, and tomato on one slice, sprinkle with salt and pepper, and top with the other slice.

3.	Heat a skillet to medium heat, and drizzle ½ teaspoon of the olive oil before putting the sandwich in the skillet.

4.   Cook for 3-5 minutes, then lift the sandwich with a spatula, drizzle the remaining ½ teaspoon olive oil into the skillet, and flip the sandwich to grill the other side for 3-5 minutes.

5.   Finish and Serve

6.   Press it down with the spatula to seal the vegetables inside. Once done, remove from the skillet and slice in half to serve.

7.   You can also toast the bread and assemble it as a simple sandwich, or brush the bread with olive oil, assemble the sandwich, and put in the toaster oven for 10-15 minutes at 350°F.

Nutrition Info: Per Serving: Calories 322; Total fat: 14g; Carbs: 40g; Fiber: 11g; Protein: 12g

Pesto Pearled Barley

Servings: 4

Cooking Time: 50 Minutes

Ingredients:

- 1 cup dried barley
- 2½ cups vegetable broth
- ½ cup Parm-y Kale Pesto

Directions:

1. Preparing the Ingredients.

2. In a medium saucepan, combine the barley and broth, then bring to boil.

3. Cover, reduce the heat to low, and simmer for about 45 minutes until tender.

4. Remove from the stove and let it stand for 5 minutes.

5. Finish and Serve

6. Fluff the barley, then gently fold in the pesto.

7. Scoop about ¾ cup into each of 4 single-compartment storage containers. Let it cool before sealing the lids.

Nutrition Info: Per Serving: Calories: 237; Fat: 6g; Protein: 9g; Carbohydrates: 40g; Fiber: 11g; Sugar: 2g; Sodium: 365mg

Brown Rice, Broccoli, and Walnut

Servings: 4

Cooking Time: 18 Minutes

Ingredients:

- 1 cup of brown rice
- 1 medium white onion, peeled, chopped
- 1 pound broccoli florets
- ½ cup chopped walnuts, toasted
- ½ teaspoon minced garlic
- ⅛ teaspoon ground black pepper
- ½ teaspoon salt
- 1 tablespoon vegan butter
- 1 cup vegetable broth
- 1 cup shredded vegan cheddar cheese

Directions:

1.   Take a saucepan, place it over medium heat, add butter and when it melts, add onion and garlic and cook for 3 minutes.

2.   Stir in rice, pour in the broth, bring the mixture to boil, then switch heat to medium-low level and simmer until rice has absorbed all the liquid.

3.   Meanwhile, take a casserole dish, place broccoli florets in it, sprinkle with salt and black pepper, cover

with a plastic wrap and microwave for 5 minutes until tender.

4.   Place cooked rice in a dish, top with broccoli, sprinkle with nuts and cheese, and then serve.

Nutrition Info: Calories: 368 Cal; Fat: 23 g: Carbs: 30.4 g; Protein: 15.1 g; Fiber: 5.7 g

Brown Rice Pilaf

Servings: 4

Cooking Time: 25 Minutes

Ingredients:

- 1 cup cooked chickpeas
- 3/4 cup brown rice, cooked
- 1/4 cup chopped cashews
- 2 cups sliced mushrooms
- 2 carrots, sliced
- ½ teaspoon minced garlic
- 1 1/2 cups chopped white onion
- 3 tablespoons vegan butter
- ½ teaspoon salt
- ¼ teaspoon ground black pepper
- 1/4 cup chopped parsley

Directions:

1.   Take a large skillet pan, place it over medium heat, add butter and when it melts, add onions and cook them for 5 minutes until softened.

2.   Then add carrots and garlic, cook for 5 minutes, add mushrooms, cook for 10 minutes until browned, add chickpeas and cook for another minute.

3.   When done, remove the pan from heat, add nuts, parsley, salt and black pepper, toss until mixed, and garnish with parsley.

4.   Serve straight away.

Nutrition Info: Calories: 409 Ca; Fat: 17.1 g: Carbs: 54 g; Protein: 12.5 g; Fiber: 6.7 g

Coconut Chickpea Curry

Servings: 4

Cooking Time: 30 Minutes

Ingredients:

- 2 teaspoons coconut flour
- 16 ounces cooked chickpeas
- 14 ounces tomatoes, diced
- 1 large red onion, sliced
- 1 ½ teaspoon minced garlic
- ½ teaspoon of sea salt
- 1 teaspoon curry powder
- 1/3 teaspoon ground black pepper
- 1 ½ tablespoons garam masala
- 1/4 teaspoon cumin
- 1 small lime, juiced
- 13.5 ounces coconut milk, unsweetened
- 2 tablespoons coconut oil

Directions:

1. Take a large pot, place it over medium-high heat, add oil and when it melts, add onions and tomatoes, season with salt and black pepper and cook for 5 minutes.

2.   Switch heat to medium-low level, cook for 10 minutes until tomatoes have released their liquid, then add chickpeas and stir in garlic, curry powder, garam masala, and cumin until combined.

3.   Stir in milk and flour, bring the mixture to boil, then switch heat to medium heat and simmer the curry for 12 minutes until cooked.

4.   Taste to adjust seasoning, drizzle with lime juice, and serve.

Nutrition Info: Calories: 225 Cal; Fat: 9.4 g: Carbs: 28.5 g; Protein: 7.3 g; Fiber: 9 g

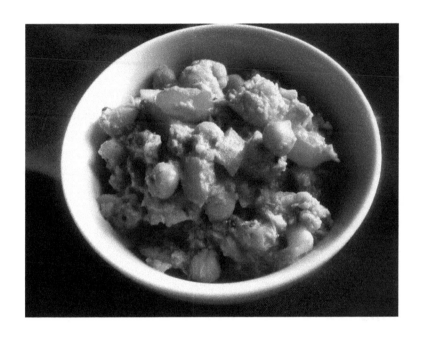

Balsamic Black Beans

Servings: 5

Cooking Time: 20 Minutes

Ingredients:

- 1 teaspoon extra-virgin olive oil or vegetable broth
- ½ cup diced sweet onion
- 1 teaspoon ground cumin
- 1 teaspoon ground cardamom (optional)
- 2 (14.5-ounce) cans black beans, rinsed and drained
- ¼ to ½ cup vegetable broth
- 2 tablespoons balsamic vinegar

Directions:

1. Preparing the Ingredients

2. In a large pot over medium-high heat, heat the olive oil.

3. Add the onion, cumin, and cardamom (if using) and sauté for 5 minutes until the onion is translucent. Add the beans and ¼ cup broth, then bring to boil. Add up to ½ cup more of broth for "soupier" beans.

4.   Cover, reduce the heat, then simmer for 10 minutes. Add the balsamic vinegar, increase the heat to medium-high, and cook for 3 more minutes uncovered.

5.   Finish and Serve

6.   Transfer to a large storage container, or divide the beans evenly among 5 single-serving storage containers. Let it cool before sealing the lids.

7.   Place the airtight containers in the refrigerator for up to 5 days, or freeze for up to 2 months. To thaw, refrigerate overnight. Reheat in the microwave for 1½-3 minutes.

Nutrition Info: Per Serving: Calories: 200; Fat: 2g; Protein: 13g; Carbohydrates: 34g; Fiber: 12g; Sugar: 1g; Sodium: 41mg

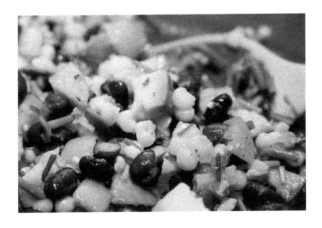

Garlic And White Bean Soup

Servings: 4

Cooking Time: 10 Minutes

Ingredients:

- 45 ounces cooked cannellini beans
- 1/4 teaspoon dried thyme
- 2 teaspoons minced garlic
- 1/8 teaspoon crushed red pepper
- 1/2 teaspoon dried rosemary
- 1/8 teaspoon ground black pepper
- 2 tablespoons olive oil
- 4 cups vegetable broth

Directions:

1.   Place one-third of white beans in a food processor, then pour in 2 cups broth and pulse for 2 minutes until smooth.

2.   Place a pot over medium heat, add oil and when hot, add garlic and cook for 1 minute until fragrant.

3.   Add pureed beans into the pan along with remaining beans, sprinkle with spices and herbs, pour in the broth, stir until combined, and bring the mixture to boil over medium-high heat.

4.   Switch heat to medium-low level, simmer the beans for 15 minutes, and then mash them with a fork.

5.   Taste the soup to adjust seasoning and then serve.

Nutrition Info: Calories: 222 Cal; Fat: 7 g: Carbs: 13 g; Protein: 11.2 g; Fiber: 9.1 g

Quinoa and Chickpeas Salad

Servings: 4

Cooking Time: 0 Minute

Ingredients:

- 3/4 cup chopped broccoli
- 1/2 cup quinoa, cooked
- 15 ounces cooked chickpeas
- ½ teaspoon minced garlic
- 1/3 teaspoon ground black pepper
- 2/3 teaspoon salt
- 1 teaspoon dried tarragon
- 2 teaspoons mustard
- 1 tablespoon lemon juice
- 3 tablespoons olive oil

Directions:

1. Take a large bowl, place all the ingredients in it, and stir until well combined.

2. Serve straight away.

Nutrition Info: Calories: 264 Cal; Fat: 12.3 g: Carbs: 32 g; Protein: 7.1 g; Fiber: 5.1 g

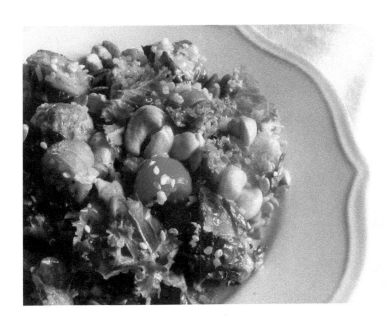

Five-spice Farro

Servings: 4

Cooking Time: 35 Minutes

Ingredients:

- 1 cup dried farro, rinsed and drained
- 1 teaspoon five-spice powder

Directions:

1. Preparing the Ingredients

2. In a medium pot, combine the farro, five-spice powder, and enough water to cover.

3. Bring to a boil; reduce the heat to medium-low, and simmer for minutes. Drain off any excess water.

4. Finish and Serve

5. Transfer to a large storage container, or scoop 1 cup farro into each of 4 storage containers. Let cool before sealing the lids.

6. Place the airtight containers in the refrigerator for 1 week or freeze for up to 3 months. To thaw, refrigerate overnight. Reheat in the microwave for 1½ to 3 minutes.

Nutrition Info: Per Serving: Calories: 73; Fat: 0g; Protein: 3g; Carbohydrates: 15g; Fiber: 1g; Sugar: 0g; Sodium: 0mg

Pineapple Fried Rice

Servings: 2

Cooking Time: 12 Minutes

Ingredients:

- 2 cups brown rice, cooked
- 1/2 cup sunflower seeds, toasted
- 2/3 cup green peas
- 1 teaspoon minced garlic
- 1 large red bell pepper, cored, diced
- 1 tablespoon grated ginger
- 2/3 cup pineapple chunks with juice
- 2 tablespoons coconut oil
- 1 bunch of green onions, sliced
- For the Sauce:
- 4 tablespoons soy sauce
- 1/2 cup pineapple juice
- 1/2 teaspoon sesame oil
- 1/2 a lime, juiced

Directions:

1.   Take a skillet pan, place it over medium-high heat, add oil and when hot, add red bell pepper, pineapple

pieces, and two-third of onion, cook for 5 minutes, then stir in ginger and garlic and cook for minute.

2.   Switch heat to the high level, add rice to the pan, stir until combined and cook for 5 minutes.

3.   When done, fold in sunflower seeds and peas and set aside until required.

4.   Prepare the sauce and for this, place sesame oil in a small bowl, add soy sauce and pineapple juice and whisk until combined.

5.   Drizzle sauce over rice, drizzle with lime juice, and serve straight away.

Nutrition Info: Calories: 179 Cal; Fat: 5.5 g: Carbs: 30 g; Protein: 3.3 g; Fiber: 2 g

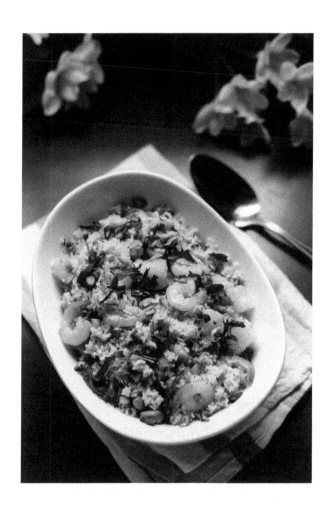

Falafel

Servings: 4

Cooking Time: 30 Minutes

Ingredients:

- ¼ cup and 1 tablespoon olive oil
- 1 cup chickpeas, cooked
- ½ cup chopped parsley
- ½ cup chopped red onion
- ½ cup chopped cilantro
- 2 teaspoons minced garlic
- ½ teaspoon ground black pepper
- ¼ teaspoon ground cinnamon
- 1 teaspoon of sea salt
- ½ teaspoon ground cumin

Directions:

1. Place all the ingredients in a food processor, reserving ¼ cup oil, and pulse until smooth.
2. Shape the mixture into small patties, place them on a rimmed baking sheet, greased with remaining oil and bake for 30 minutes until cooked and roasted on both sides, turning halfway through.
3. Serve straight away.

Nutrition Info: Calories: 354 Cal; Fat: 20.7 g: Carbs: 34.6 g; Protein: 11 g; Fiber: 7 g

Lemon And Thyme Couscous

Servings: 6

Cooking Time: 10 Minutes

Ingredients:

- 2¾ cups vegetable stock
- juice and zest of 1 lemon
- 2 tablespoons chopped fresh thyme
- 1½ cups couscous
- ¼ cup chopped fresh parsley
- sea salt
- freshly ground black pepper

Directions:

1.   Preparing the Ingredients

2.   In a medium pot, bring the vegetable stock, lemon juice, and thyme to a boil. Stir in the couscous, cover, and remove from the heat.

3.   Allow to sit, covered, until the -couscous absorbs the liquid and softens, about 5 minutes. Fluff with a fork.

4.   Finish and Serve

5.   Stir in the lemon zest and parsley. Season with salt and pepper. Serve hot.

Vegan Pho
Servings: 6

Cooking Time: 15 Minutes

Ingredients:

- 1 package of wide rice noodles, cooked
- 1 medium white onion, peeled, quartered
- 2 teaspoons minced garlic
- 1 inch of ginger, sliced into coins
- 8 cups vegetable broth
- 3 whole cloves
- 2 tablespoons soy sauce
- 3 whole star anise
- 1 cinnamon stick
- 3 cups of water
- For Toppings:
- Basil as needed for topping
- Chopped green onions as needed for topping
- Ming beans as needed for topping
- Hot sauce as needed for topping
- Lime wedges for serving

Directions:

1.   Take a large pot, place it over medium-high heat, add all the ingredients for soup in it, except for soy sauce and broth, and bring it to boil.

2.   Then switch heat to medium-low level, simmer the soup for 30 minutes and then stir in soy sauce.

3.   When done, distribute cooked noodles into bowls, top with soup, then top with toppings and serve.

Nutrition Info: Calories: 31 Cal; Fat: 0 g: Carbs: 7 g; Protein: 0 g; Fiber: 2 g

Lentil Soup
Servings: 4

Cooking Time: 25 Minutes

Ingredients:
- 1 tbsp. Olive Oil
- 4 cups Vegetable Stock
- 1 Onion, finely chopped
- 2 Carrots, medium
- 1 cup Lentils, dried
- 1 tsp. Cumin

Directions:
1.   To make this healthy soup, first, you need to heat the oil in a medium-sized skillet over medium heat.

2.   Once the oil becomes hot, stir in the cumin and then the onions.

3.   Sauté them for minutes or until the onion is slightly transparent and cooked.

4.   To this, add the carrots and toss them well.

5.   Next, stir in the lentils. Mix well.

6.   Now, pour in the vegetable stock and give a good stir until everything comes together.

7.   As the soup mixture starts to boil, reduce the heat and allow it to simmer for 10 minutes while keeping the pan covered.

8.   Turn off the heat and then transfer the mixture to a bowl.

9.   Finally, blend it with an immersion blender or in a high-speed blender for 1 minute or until you get a rich, smooth mixture.

10.   Serve it hot and enjoy.

Mediterranean Vegetable Stew

Servings: 4

Cooking Time: 45 Minutes

Ingredients:

- 1 tablespoon extra-virgin olive oil
- 1 medium yellow onion, chopped
- 1 medium carrot, chopped
- 3 garlic cloves, minced
- 1 medium red bell pepper, cut into ½-inch dice
- 1 medium fennel bulb, quartered and cut into 1/4-inch slices
- 1 medium zucchini, chopped
- 1 (14.5-ounce) can diced tomatoes, undrained
- 1 cup vegetable broth
- Freshly ground black pepper
- 8 ounces white or porcini mushrooms, lightly rinsed, patted dry, and sliced
- 3 cups fresh baby spinach
- 1½ cups cooked or 1 (15.5-ounce) can cannellini beans, drained and rinsed
- ½ teaspoon dried basil
- ½ teaspoon dried marjoram
- 2 tablespoons minced fresh parsley

Directions:

1.   Preparing the Ingredients

2.   In a large saucepan, heat the oil over medium heat. Add the onion, carrot, garlic, and bell pepper. Cover and cook until softened for 7 minutes.

3.   Add the fennel, zucchini, tomatoes, and broth. Bring to a boil, then reduce heat to low. Season with salt and black pepper, cover, and simmer until the vegetables are tender for about minutes.

4.   Finish and Serve

5.   Stir in the mushrooms, spinach, beans, basil, marjoram, and parsley. Taste and adjust seasonings if necessary. Simmer for another 10 minutes. Serve immediately.

Mexican Fideo Soup with Pinto Beans

Servings: 4

Cooking Time: 25 Minutes

Ingredients:

- 3 tablespoons extra-virgin olive oil
- 1 medium onion, chopped
- 3 garlic cloves, chopped
- 8 ounces fideo, vermicelli, or angel hair pasta, broken into 2-inch pieces
- 1 (14.5-ounce) can crushed tomatoes
- 1½ cups cooked or 1 (15.5-ounce) can pinto beans, rinsed and drained
- 1 (4-ounce) can chopped hot or mild green chiles
- 1 teaspoon ground cumin
- ½ teaspoon dried oregano
- 6 cups vegetable broth, homemade (see Light Vegetable Broth) or store-bought, or water
- Salt and freshly ground black pepper
- ¼ cup chopped fresh cilantro, for garnish

Directions:

1. Preparing the Ingredients

2.   In a large soup pot, heat 1 tablespoon of oil over medium heat. Add the onion, cover, and cook until soft for about 10 minutes. Stir in the garlic and cook 1 minute longer. Remove the onion mixture with a slotted spoon and set aside.

3.   In the same pot, heat the remaining 2 tablespoons of oil over medium heat, add the noodles, and cook until golden, stirring frequently for 5 to 7 minutes. Be careful not to burn the noodles.

4.   Finish and serve.

5.   Stir in the tomatoes, beans, chiles, cumin, oregano, broth, and salt and pepper. Stir in the onion mixture and simmer until the vegetables and noodles are tender, for 10 to 1minutes. Ladle into soup bowls, garnish with cilantro, then serve.

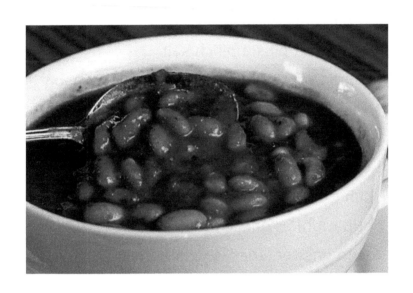

Creamy Garlic-spinach Rotini Soup

Servings: 4

Cooking Time: 15 Minutes

Ingredients:

- 1 teaspoon extra-virgin olive oil
- 1 cup chopped mushrooms
- ¼ teaspoon plus a pinch salt
- 4 garlic cloves, minced, or 1 teaspoon garlic powder
- 2 peeled carrots or ½ red bell pepper, chopped
- 6 cups Vegetable Broth or water
- Pinch freshly ground black pepper
- 1 cup rotini or gnocchi
- ¾ cup unsweetened nondairy milk
- ¼ cup nutritional yeast
- 2 cups chopped fresh spinach
- ¼ cup pitted black olives or sun-dried tomatoes, chopped
- Herbed Croutons, for topping (optional)

Directions:

1. Preparing the Ingredients

2.	Heat the olive oil in a large soup pot over medium-high heat.

3.	Add the mushrooms and a pinch of salt. Sauté for about 4 minutes until the mushrooms soften. Add the garlic (if using fresh) and carrots, then sauté for 1 minute. Add the vegetable broth, then add the remaining ¼ teaspoon of salt, and pepper (plus the garlic powder if using). Bring to boil and add the pasta. Cook for about 10 minutes until the pasta is cooked.

4.	Finish and Serve

5.	Turn off the heat and stir in the milk, nutritional yeast, spinach, and olives. Top with croutons (if using). Leftovers will keep in an airtight container for up to 1 week in the refrigerator, or up to 1 month in the freezer.

Nutrition Info: Per Serving: (2 cups) Calories 207; Protein: 11g; Total fat: 5g; Saturated fat: 1g; Carbohydrates: 34g; Fiber: 7g

Mustard Green & Potato Soup

Servings: 6

Cooking Time: 30 Minutes

Ingredients:

- 2 tbsp olive oil
- 1 red onion, chopped
- 1 leek, white part only, chopped
- 2 garlic cloves, minced
- 6 cups vegetable broth
- 1 pound red potatoes, chopped
- 1 lb sweet potatoes, diced
- ¼ tsp crushed red pepper
- 1 bunch mustard greens, chopped

Directions:

1. Heat the oil in a pot over medium heat. Place onion, leek and garlic and sauté for 5 minutes. Pour in broth, potatoes and red pepper. Bring to a boil, then lower the heat and season with salt and pepper. Simmer for minutes. Add in mustard greens, cook for 5 minutes until the greens are tender. Serve.

Hot & Sour Tofu Soup

Servings: 3

Cooking Time: 15 Minutes

Ingredients:

- 6 to 7 ounces firm or extra-firm tofu
- 1 teaspoon extra-virgin olive oil
- 1 cup sliced mushrooms
- 1 cup finely chopped cabbage
- 1 garlic clove, minced
- ½-inch piece fresh ginger, peeled and minced
- Salt
- 4 cups water or Vegetable Broth
- 2 tablespoons rice vinegar or apple cider vinegar
- 2 tablespoons soy sauce
- 1 teaspoon toasted sesame oil
- 1 teaspoon sugar
- Pinch red pepper flakes
- 1 scallion, white and light green parts only, chopped

Directions:

1. Preparing the Ingredients

2.   Press your tofu before you start: Put it between several layers of paper towels and place a heavy pan or book (with a waterproof cover or protected with plastic wrap) on top. Let it stand for 30 minutes. Discard the paper towels. Cut the tofu into ½-inch cubes.

3.   In a large soup pot, heat the olive oil over medium-high heat.

4.   Add the mushrooms, cabbage, garlic, ginger, and a pinch of salt. Sauté for 7 to 8 minutes until the vegetables are softened.

5.   Add the water, vinegar, soy sauce, sesame oil, sugar, red pepper flakes, and tofu.

6.   Bring to a boil, then turn the heat to low.

7.   Finish and Serve

8.   Simmer the soup for 5 to 10 minutes.

9.   Serve with the scallion sprinkled on top.

10.   Leftovers will keep in an airtight container for up to 1 week in the refrigerator, or up to 1 month in the freezer.

Nutrition Info: Per Serving: (2 cups) Calories 161; Protein: 13g; Total fat: 9g; Saturated fat: 1g; Carbohydrates: 10g; Fiber: 3g

Kale White Bean Soup

Servings: 4

Cooking Time: 45 Minutes

Ingredients:

- 1 Onion, medium & finely sliced
- 3 cups Kale, coarsely chopped
- 2 tsp. Olive Oil
- 15 oz. White Beans
- 4 cups Vegetable Broth
- 4 Garlic Cloves, minced
- Sea Salt & Pepper, as needed
- 2 tsp. Rosemary, fresh & chopped
- 1 lb. White Potatoes, cubed

Directions:

1. Begin by taking a large saucepan and heat it over a medium-high heat.
2. Once the pan becomes hot, spoon in the oil.
3. Next, stir in the onion and sauté for 8 to 9 minutes or until the onions are cooked and lightly browned.
4. Then, add the garlic and rosemary to the pan.
5. Sauté for a further minute or until aromatic.

6.   Now, pour in the broth along with the potatoes, black pepper, and salt. Mix well.

7.   Bring the mixture to a boil, and when it starts boiling, lower the heat.

8.   Allow it to simmer for 32 to 35 minutes or until the potatoes are cooked and tender.

9.   After that, mash the potatoes slightly by using the back of the spoon.

10.   Finally, add the kale and beans to the soup and cook for 8 minutes or until the kale is wilted.

11.   Check the seasoning. Add more salt and pepper if needed.

12.   Serve hot.

Hearty Winter Quinoa Soup
Servings: 4

Cooking Time: 25 Minutes

Ingredients:

- 2 tablespoons olive oil
- 1 onion, chopped
- 2 carrots, peeled and chopped
- 1 parsnip, chopped
- 1 celery stalk, chopped
- 1 cup yellow squash, chopped
- 4 garlic cloves, pressed or minced
- 4 cups roasted vegetable broth
- 2 medium tomatoes, crushed
- 1 cup quinoa
- Sea salt and ground black pepper, to taste
- 1 bay laurel
- 2 cup Swiss chard, tough ribs removed and torn into pieces
- 2 tablespoons Italian parsley, chopped

Directions:

1.   In a heavy-bottomed pot, heat the olive over medium-high heat. Now, sauté the onion, carrot,

parsnip, celery and yellow squash for about 3 minutes or until the vegetables are just tender.

2.   Add in the garlic and continue to sauté for 1 minute or until aromatic.

3.   Then, stir in the vegetable broth, tomatoes, quinoa, salt, pepper and bay laurel; bring to a boil. Immediately reduce the heat to a simmer and let it cook for 1minutes.

4.   Fold in the Swiss chard; continue to simmer until the chard wilts.

5.   Ladle into individual bowls and serve garnished with the fresh parsley. Bon appétit!

Nutrition Info: Per Serving: Calories: 328; Fat: 11.1g; Carbs: 44.1g; Protein: 13.3g

Spicy Bean Stew
Servings: 4

Cooking Time: 50 Minutes

Ingredients:

- 7 ounces cooked black eye beans
- 14 ounces chopped tomatoes
- 2 medium carrots, peeled, diced
- 7 ounces cooked kidney beans
- 1 leek, diced
- ½ a chili, chopped
- 1 teaspoon minced garlic
- 1/3 teaspoon ground black pepper
- 2/3 teaspoon salt
- 1 teaspoon red chili powder
- 1 lemon, juiced
- 3 tablespoons white wine
- 1 tablespoon olive oil
- 1 2/3 cups vegetable stock

Directions:

1.   Take a large saucepan, place it over medium-high heat, add oil and when hot, add leeks and cook for 8 minutes or until softened.

2.	Then add carrots, continue cooking for 4 minutes, stir in chili and garlic, pour in the wine, and continue cooking for minutes.

3.	Add tomatoes, stir in lemon juice, pour in the stock and bring the mixture to boil.

4.	Switch heat to medium level, simmer for 35 minutes until stew has thickened, then add both beans along with remaining ingredients and cook for 5 minutes until hot.

5.	Serve straight away.

Nutrition Info: Calories: 114 Cal; Fat: 1.6 g: Carbs: 19 g; Protein: 6 g; Fiber: 8.4 g

Noodle Soup

Servings: 6

Cooking Time: 30 Minutes

Ingredients:

- 2 tbsp olive oil
- 1 onion, chopped
- 1 carrot, sliced
- 2 garlic cloves, minced
- 1 (28-oz) can crushed tomatoes
- 1 cup Chana dal, rinsed, and drained
- 1 tsp dried thyme
- 6 cups vegetable broth
- 4 oz soba noodles, broken into thirds

Directions:

1.   Warm the oil in a pot over medium heat. Place in onion, carrot and garlic and sauté for 5 minutes. Add in tomatoes, chana dal, thyme, and broth. Bring to a boil, then lower the heat and season with salt and pepper. Simmer for minutes. Stir in soba noodles, cook 5 minutes more. Serve immediately.

Classic Vegan Coleslaw

Servings: 4

Cooking Time: 10 Minutes

Ingredients:

- 1 pound red cabbage, shredded
- 2 carrots, trimmed and grated
- 4 tablespoons onion, chopped
- 1 garlic clove, minced
- 1/2 cup fresh Italian parsley, roughly chopped
- 1 cup vegan mayo
- 1 teaspoon brown mustard
- 1 teaspoon lemon zest
- 2 tablespoons apple cider vinegar
- Sea salt and ground black pepper, to taste
- 2 tablespoons sunflower seeds

Directions:

1. Toss the cabbage, carrots, onion, garlic and parsley in a salad bowl.

2. In a mixing bowl, whisk the mayo, mustard, lemon zest, apple cider vinegar, salt and black pepper.

3. Dress your salad and serve garnished with the sunflower seeds.

Nutrition Info: Per Serving: Calories: 293; Fat: 25.8g; Carbs: 14g; Protein: 3.5g

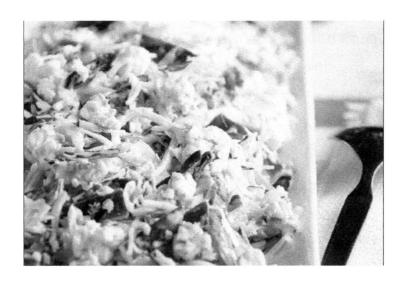

Asian-inspired Chili

Servings: 4

Cooking Time: 20 Minutes

Ingredients:

- 1 teaspoon sesame oil or 2 teaspoons vegetable broth or water
- 1 cup diced onion
- 3 teaspoons minced garlic (about 3 cloves)
- 1 cup chopped carrots
- 2 cups shredded green or napa cabbage
- 1 (14.5-ounce) can small red beans or adzuki beans, drained and rinsed
- 1 (14.5-ounce) fire-roasted diced tomatoes
- 2 cups vegetable broth
- 2 tablespoons red miso paste or tomato paste
- 2 tablespoons hot water
- 1 tablespoon hot sauce
- 2 teaspoons to 1 tablespoon tamari or soy sauce (optional)

Directions:

1.   Preparing the Ingredients

2. In a large pot, over medium-high heat, heat the sesame oil. Add the onion, garlic, and carrot. Sauté for 5 minutes until the onions are translucent. Add the cabbage, beans, tomatoes, and broth, then stir well. Bring to a boil.

3. Cover, reduce the heat to low, and simmer for 15 minutes.

4. In a measuring cup, whisk the miso paste and hot water. Set aside.

5. After 1minutes, remove the chili from the stove, add the miso mixture and hot sauce, and stir well. Taste before determining how much tamari to add (if using).

6. Finish and Serve

7. Divide the chili evenly among 4 single-serving containers or large glass jars. Let it cool before sealing the lids.

8. Place the containers in the refrigerator for up to 5 days, or freeze for up to 3 months. To thaw, refrigerate overnight. Reheat in the microwave for 2 to 3 minutes.

Nutrition Info: Per Serving: Calories: 177; Protein: 9g; Total fat: 2g; Carbohydrates: 33g; Fiber: 191g

Moroccan Lentil and Raisin Salad

Servings: 4

Cooking Time: 20 Minutes

Ingredients:

- 1 cup red lentils, rinsed
- 1 large carrot, julienned
- 1 Persian cucumber, thinly sliced
- 1 sweet onion, chopped
- 1/2 cup golden raisins
- 1/4 cup fresh mint, snipped
- 1/4 cup fresh basil, snipped
- 1/4 cup extra-virgin olive oil
- 1/4 cup lemon juice, freshly squeezed
- 1 teaspoon grated lemon peel
- 1/2 teaspoon fresh ginger root, peeled and minced
- 1/2 teaspoon granulated garlic
- 1 teaspoon ground allspice
- Sea salt and ground black pepper, to taste

Directions:

1.   In a large-sized saucepan, bring 3 cups of the water and cup of the lentils to a boil.

2. Immediately turn the heat to a simmer and continue to cook your lentils for a further 15 to 17 minutes or until they've softened but are not mushy yet. Drain and let it cool completely.

3. Transfer the lentils to a salad bowl; add in the carrot, cucumber and sweet onion. Then, add the raisins, mint and basil to your salad.

4. In a small mixing dish, whisk the olive oil, lemon juice, lemon peel, ginger, granulated garlic, allspice, salt and black pepper.

5. Dress your salad and serve well-chilled. Bon appétit!

Nutrition Info: Per Serving: Calories: 418; Fat: 15g; Carbs: 62.9g; Protein: 12.4g

White Bean and Cabbage Stew

Servings: 4

Cooking Time: 8 Hours

Ingredients:

- 3 cups cooked great northern beans
- 1.5 pounds potatoes, peeled, cut in large dice
- 1 large white onion, peeled, chopped
- ½ head of cabbage, chopped
- 3 ribs celery, chopped
- 4 medium carrots, peeled, sliced
- 14.5 ounces diced tomatoes
- 1/3 cup pearled barley
- 1 teaspoon minced garlic
- ½ teaspoon ground black pepper
- 1 bay leaf
- 1 teaspoon dried thyme
- ½ teaspoon crushed rosemary
- 1 teaspoon salt
- ½ teaspoon caraway seeds
- 1 tablespoon chopped parsley
- 8 cups vegetable broth

Directions:

1.   Switch on the slow cooker, then add all the ingredients except for salt, parsley, tomatoes, and beans and stir until mixed.

2.   Shut the slow cooker with lid, and cook for 7 hours at low heat setting until cooked.

3.   Then stir in remaining ingredients, stir until combined and continue cooking for 1 hour.

4.   Serve straight away

Nutrition Info: Calories: 150 Cal; Fat: 0.7 g: Carbs: 27 g; Protein: 7 g; Fiber: 9.4 g

Coconut Artichoke Soup with Almonds

Servings: 4

Cooking Time: 30 Minutes

Ingredients:

- 1 tbsp olive oil
- 2 medium shallots, chopped
- 2 (10-oz) packages artichoke hearts
- 3 cups vegetable broth
- 1 tsp fresh lemon juice
- Salt to taste
- ⅓ cup plant butter
- ⅛ tsp ground cayenne pepper
- 1 cup plain coconut cream
- 1 tbsp snipped fresh chives
- 2 tbsp sliced toasted almonds

Directions:

1.   Heat the oil in a pot over medium heat. Place in shallots and sauté until softened, about 3 minutes. Add in artichokes, broth, lemon juice, and salt. Bring to a boil, lower the heat, and simmer for minutes. Stir in butter and cayenne pepper. Transfer to a food processor and blend until purée. Return to the pot. Mix in the coconut

cream and simmer for 5 minutes. Serve topped with chives and almonds.

Coconut Mushroom Soup

Servings: 2

Cooking Time: 20 Minutes

Ingredients:

- 2 tsp olive oil
- 1 onion, chopped
- 2 garlic cloves, minced
- 2 cups chopped mushrooms
- Salt and black pepper to taste
- 2 tbsp whole-wheat flour
- 1 tsp dried rosemary
- 4 cups vegetable broth
- 1 cup coconut cream

Directions:

1. In a pot over medium heat, warm the oil. Place the onion, garlic, mushrooms, and salt and cook for 5 minutes. Stir in the flour and cook for another 2 minutes. Add in rosemary, vegetable broth, coconut cream, and pepper. Lower the heat and simmer for 10 minutes. Serve.

Fall Medley Stew

Servings: 4

Cooking Time: 65 Minutes

Ingredients:

- 2 tbsp olive oil
- 8 oz seitan, cubed
- 1 leek, chopped
- 2 garlic cloves, minced
- 1 russet potato, chopped
- 1 carrot, chopped
- 1 parsnip, chopped
- 1 cup butternut squash, cubed
- 1 head savoy cabbage, chopped
- 1 (14.5-oz) can diced tomatoes
- 1 (15.5-oz) can white beans
- 2 cups vegetable broth
- ½ cup dry white wine
- ½ tsp dried thyme
- ½ cup crumbled angel hair pasta

Directions:

1.   Heat oil in a pot over medium heat. Place in seitan and cook for 3 minutes. Sprinkle with salt and pepper.

Add in leek and garlic and cook for another 3 minutes. Stir in potato, carrot, parsnip, and squash, cook for minutes. Add in cabbage, tomatoes, white beans, broth, wine, thyme, salt, and pepper. Bring to a boil, lower the heat and simmer for 15 minutes. Put in pasta and cook for 5 minutes.

Thai-style Tempeh and Noodle Salad

Servings: 3

Cooking Time: 45 Minutes

Ingredients:

- 6 ounces tempeh
- 4 tablespoons rice vinegar
- 4 tablespoons soy sauce
- 2 garlic cloves, minced
- 1 small-sized lime, freshly juiced
- 5 ounces rice noodles
- 1 carrot, julienned
- 1 shallot, chopped
- 3 handfuls Chinese cabbage, thinly sliced
- 3 handfuls kale, torn into pieces
- 1 bell pepper, seeded and thinly sliced
- 1 bird's eye chili, minced
- 1/4 cup peanut butter
- 2 tablespoons agave syrup

Directions:

1.   Place the tempeh, 2 tablespoons of the rice vinegar, soy sauce, garlic and lime juice in a ceramic dish; let it marinate for about 40 minutes.

103

2.   Meanwhile, cook the rice noodles according to the package directions. Drain your noodles and transfer them to a salad bowl.

3.   Add the carrot, shallot, cabbage, kale and peppers to the salad bowl. Add in the peanut butter, the remaining 2 tablespoons of the rice vinegar and agave syrup and toss to combine well.

4.   Top with the marinated tempeh and serve immediately. Enjoy!

Nutrition Info: Per Serving: Calories: 494; Fat: 14.5g; Carbs: 75g; Protein: 18.7g

Root Vegetable Bisque

Servings: 4 To 6

Cooking Time: 35 Minutes

Ingredients:

- 1 tablespoon extra-virgin olive oil
- 3 large shallots, chopped
- 2 large carrots, shredded
- 2 medium parsnips, shredded
- 1 medium potato, peeled and chopped
- 2 garlic cloves, minced
- ½ teaspoon dried thyme
- ¼ teaspoon dried marjoram
- 4 cups vegetable broth, or store-bought, or water
- 1 cup plain unsweetened soy milk
- Salt and freshly ground black pepper
- 1 tablespoon minced fresh parsley, garnish

Directions:

1. Preparing the Ingredients

2. In a large soup pot, heat the oil over medium heat. Add the shallots, carrots, parsnips, potato, and garlic. Cover and cook until softened for about 5 minutes. Add the thyme, marjoram, and broth and bring to boil.

Reduce heat to low and simmer, uncovered, until the vegetables are tender for about 30 minutes.

3.   Finish and Serve

4.   Purée the soup in the pot with an immersion blender or food processor in batches if necessary, then return to the pot. Stir in the soy milk and taste, adjusting the seasoning if necessary. Heat the soup over low heat until hot. Ladle into bowls, sprinkle with parsley, then serve.

Cayenne Pumpkin Soup

Servings: 6

Cooking Time: 55 Minutes

Ingredients:

- 1 (2 pounds) pumpkin, sliced
- 3 tbsp olive oil
- 1 tsp salt
- 2 red bell peppers
- 1 onion, halved
- 1 head garlic
- 6 cups water
- Zest and juice of 1 lime
- ¼ tsp cayenne pepper
- ½ tsp ground coriander
- ½ tsp ground cumin
- Toasted pumpkin seeds

Directions:

1.   Preheat oven to 350 F.

2.   Brush the pumpkin slices with oil and sprinkle with salt.

3.   Arrange the slices skin side-down and on a greased baking dish and bake for 20 minutes. Brush the

107

onion with oil. Cut the top of garlic head and brush with oil.

4.	When the pumpkin is done, add in bell peppers, onion and garlic, and bake for another 10 minutes. Allow to cool.

5.	Take out the flesh from the pumpkin skin and transfer to a food processor. Cut the pepper roughly, peel and cut the onion, and remove the cloves from the garlic head. Transfer to the food processor and pour in the water, lime zest and lime juice.

6.	Blend the soup until smooth. If it's very thick, add a bit of water to reach your desired consistency. Sprinkle with salt, cayenne, coriander, and cumin. Serve.

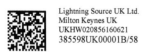